PSORIASIS, HEALING FROM THE INSIDE OUT

PSORIASIS, HEALING FROM THE INSIDE OUT

*A personal story of triumph over the disease
psoriasis and an awakening of the notion that we
are indeed in charge of our own healing.*

HEATHER J. FERRIS

Cover design and illustrations
by Peggy Reine Cromer

*Everywhere I go, I meet people who want to be
fully well, who are tired of feeling overwhelmed,
and who are yearning to take charge of their lives.*

JOHN ROBBINS,
  In Search of Balance and *Diet for a New America*

This book is dedicated to all psoriasis
sufferers, who are tired of psoriasis controlling
  their lives.
It is time to end the suffering and heartbreak
and get on with the healing.

HEATHER J. FERRIS

TABLE OF CONTENTS

❦

PART ONE

❦

PART TWO

🌿

ACKNOWLEDGEMENTS

There are many people who have supported me in my quest for healing. I would like to especially thank my parents Inez and Charles Ferris for their love, encouragement and belief in life. Many thanks to my daughters Kirstie, Wendy and Robyn, my siblings, Brian, Margaret, Shirley, Jenny and my friends around the world who loved me despite the psoriasis. They obviously knew more about my inner beauty than I did! A special appreciation to Margaret Rice who was always my friend and who followed her intuition and sent me the Linotar product when I was ready for it. I appreciate the encouragement and letters of support from my hairstylist Diane; Tricia, a wonderful massage therapist; and Dr Stuart Brown; all of whom attest to the remarkable healing that has taken place.

I would like to acknowledge the following people for their contributions:

My friend and initial editor, Myrette Drummond who has a knack for the English language and is so respectful of me and my story.

Jack Canfield of Self-Esteem Seminars CA who gave us permission to include the Total Truth Process.

Donna Martin for permission to use the exercise, Inner Smiling.

Dr Len Walt and Dr Steve Faulkner who read my work and were very encouraging.

Maxine Carpenter for her feedback.

Peggy Reine Cromer, my friend and the graphic artist who did a great job. We had many laughs.

My deepest gratitude goes to my publisher, affectionately known as "White feather" for her tireless work on my behalf.

INTRODUCTION

*Because a thing seems difficult for you, do not
think it is impossible for anyone to accomplish. But
whatever is possible for another, believe that you,
too, are capable of it.*

MARCUS AURELIUS ANTONINUS

I sit here on a warm afternoon in Qualicum Beach, British
Columbia, Canada, wearing shorts and a shirt, my skin clear
and brown. I feel more peaceful, content and blessed. This is
quite different from last July and probably thirty Julys before
this one. It is quite possible I would have been sitting here
scratching my scalp unconsciously, staring at the large red
lesions on my legs and arms, reminders of the disease that has
taken so much of my time and energy for so long.

I was seventeen when I first developed psoriasis. It appeared first in my armpits and then quickly spread. My worst
fears were confirmed. Body image had always been a problem
for me. I thought I was fat. In fact I believed that when people looked at me, all they saw was this fat body. The idea that
they would now see me as a patchy, red, diseased fat body was
more than I could bear.

I was hopeful (more like desperate) at first, that the medication would cure it, but as time passed I realized that psori-

asis was in control. I began to see psoriasis as something real, in its own right, not the effect of something inside. I would talk about 'my' psoriasis as I allowed it to become part of me.

The family I was born into was/is quite unusual, in that my parents believed in healing in a holistic way. There is a strong spiritual base to their belief system, though standard and alternative treatments have their place too. They watched my struggle with psoriasis, feeling helpless, and knowing that I was capable of healing myself in whichever way I was led. They were very supportive of anything I tried, and their belief that there is always an answer, kept me motivated to continue my search.

Many medical and alternative treatments were offered me; some helped, others didn't. The psoriasis would either improve a little and return, or not improve at all. Does this sound familiar?

Summers were easier because the psoriasis on my body healed in the sun. I would spend hours out in the sun, finding private places so as to expose more of my skin: draping sheets around balconies or lying behind bushes. As winter approached I would become quite despondent. I felt obliged to be in the sun whenever it was warm enough, even when I had more pressing things to do. I definitely felt controlled by the weather. I was feeling pretty helpless and alone, as I knew no one with psoriasis.

In the many childhood moves to new schools, I had experienced feeling different and somewhat rejected. At that time, I remember looking around at my classmates in grade seven. Sheena Bayne seemed to me to be the one girl most accepted by everyone. I noticed that she was very kind and friendly to all. She became a model for me, someone I could try to be like. It didn't occur to me that I was enough, just being myself and that my fear of not being accepted was probably causing my rejection.

I decided that the way I would deal with this new challenge of psoriasis, would be to become a really 'nice' person (like Sheena Bayne). My plan was to make eye contact with people and they would see 'me' through my eyes, and they would like me. By keeping eye contact I would stop them from looking at my body. This was what I had hoped.

Life went on despite psoriasis and it didn't really limit my life, other than the time it took and my own inner stress about it. I went to university and became a teacher, marrying around my twenty-fourth birthday.

I had been married for two years when my husband was diagnosed with a brain tumour. This was a very difficult time and my skin did not seem important compared to what he was going through. The doctors could not help Stuart, other than prescribing drugs for pain, so he chose "grape therapy". I had learned some of the importance of body/mind/spirit exercises through my parents' experience of healing. This was a time of experimentation for us. The doctors had predicted that he would die within three weeks. He lived five months and all that time, he had no headaches. He had bright eyes and mind, and a very healthy looking skin. We had obviously hoped that the tumour would somehow disappear, but that wasn't to be. In looking back, I recognized how the grape juice diet had kept so much of his body healthy.

It was important for me to be strong at this time, and I was encouraged by friends to take care of myself. I ate a very healthy diet, we meditated and did creative visualizations regularly to try to help Stuart's healing process. It helped me too. My body was free of psoriasis for the first time, returning a couple of months after his death.

I did an annual ten day grape diet/fast for two or three years after Stuart died, and each time experienced beautiful hair and skin and a feeling of inner cleanliness. In itself it is not a wonder cure for the psoriasis, but part of the cleansing process necessary for healing.

I did not grieve easily because I had always prided myself in being very strong (my belief system at the time was that crying was a sign of weakness). As a result, I carried the pain for many years, until I learned that the stress, from unresolved emotional issues, causes sickness and there are healthy ways of coping with emotional pain.

After a few years, I married again, gave birth to my first daughter and emigrated from South Africa to Canada. Immigration implies a huge change, which I took in my stride, again not admitting the cost to my system. Life on the prairies was hard. It was very cold; we had little money, five acres of land and a house to build. I had two more babies within three years, a husband who was away working seventy-five percent of the time and two goats which constantly escaped. I felt totally stressed out. Not surprisingly, the psoriasis was at its all time worst.

The psoriasis was driving me crazy. I went to yet another dermatologist. My experiences with skin specialists had not been great. I was told by one that psoriasis was the dermatologist's dream, because there was no cure. It kept them in business and their patients never died. This particular doctor looked at me with absolutely no compassion. Eighty percent of my body, from head to toe, was covered in angry lesions. I was embarrassed to have him looking at me. He never once asked me what was going on in my life. He seemed interested only in the disease, as if it was an enemy approaching that needed to be stopped at all costs.

He wrote out a prescription for methotrexate and told me to go and have my blood tested. I asked about the treatment and the side-effects. I was told I would need to have my blood checked regularly and that they would be watching my liver. I began to feel insecure. I had psoriasis. I was not sick and I had no intention of jeopardizing the health of my liver. I didn't know what to say. After all, he was the expert! My self-esteem was at an all-time low.

By the time I had dressed, I was in tears. I felt extremely vulnerable. The nurse came in and I told her that I was not prepared to go this route. She went to the doctor and came back with the message, that if I wasn't willing for him to do his job and clear my skin, there was nothing further he could do for me. I might as well use vaseline. This I did for many years.

At that point I decided to give up the medical route. It was time for me to discover the nature of psoriasis for myself, trusting that I would ultimately have some success in clearing my body. My goal was to understand what triggered psoriasis in my body.

My decision to abandon medical cures was strengthened by yet another stressful experience. A slipped disc in my spine caused me agony from sciatica. My experience again took me away from the medical route. My general practitioner found me in the hospital on the eve of my having back surgery. After we had discussed my condition, he took the time to investigate my medical report and advised me not to go into surgery. He felt that it was possible the surgeon was being a bit hasty and that a more conservative approach was needed. What a gift! After some time in physiotherapy I began to heal and I was becoming more aware of alternate therapies. I was led into yoga—"led"meaning I met someone who was a yoga instructor and my intuition said, "This makes sense."I had been advised by the doctors and physiotherapists that I would never be able to bend forward again. When I told my yoga instructor that I could do anything except bend over, she smiled and said, "We'll see". I totally recovered and could participate fully in all exercises.

These experiences together, on reflection, caused me to begin the inward journey to discover what my body was trying to teach me. I wanted to be well; I did not need disease. The idea of changing from the inside opened up a whole new world. I began to read books on psychology and personal growth. I practised yoga. I monitored both food intake and stressors to see if I could pinpoint the triggers. I went back to university to study counselling, because by now I was so intrigued by what I was learning, I wanted to work in the mental health and community education fields.

Psoriasis was no longer my main focus. I was interested in life and how we humans weave our webs. This was how I became committed to my growth and learning, which I now realize is a major purpose for my life. Part of this purpose is also helping others experience their own healing through the awareness of themselves. I have been working professionally as a counsellor/consultant and personal growth coach for the past eleven years.

It has become really clear to me what foods and stressors contribute to my experience of psoriasis. I have accepted myself and my body, which is actually quite attractive. Two years ago, I made a commitment to my health, putting to work much of what I had learned. I lost weight without dieting, made some lifestyle changes, including a regular massage, and the psoriasis lessened in intensity. I am told I look younger and I feel great!

The bonus came when I received a topical product in the mail from a dear friend in South Africa. Linotar/Exorex (gel, cream and conditioner) comes without need of a prescription, is easy to use, and excellent results are obtained when it is used in conjunction with the lifestyle changes that I am already living. After about fifteen days, I noticed a ninety-five percent improvement. Product details can be found at the back of the book. It must be stressed that any of the products on the market today will not cure psoriasis by themselves.

My healing journey has now taken me through thirty years of learning. It has taught me that becoming a nice person, one that *I* like, is a long and often painful process. The rewards and the joy far outweigh the pain, and I would have it no other way. This new way of life is leading me to a place of inner peace and happiness. I feel really fortunate. Would I have chosen this path if it hadn't been for psoriasis? I don't know. I do know that psoriasis is no longer my enemy. It is an indicator of my inner unrest and I can do something about that.

So how do you start? Only you can determine your own healing process. As you learn to listen to your body, and try out some of the following ideas, you will experience healing in the body, mind and spirit. There is no quick fix, but you can have fun on the way. Part One of this book describes psoriasis and deals with changes in diet, lifestyle and attitude. Part Two includes body and mind exercises, that will help you to change habits and create a more peaceful internal environment. I have included some of the most common medical treatments for your interest, as well as a couple of letters from psoriasis sufferers. I believe it is important to be informed and to make the choices that are best for us individually.

This book can be used for your own self-discovery and healing. It does not replace medical advice. It merely shares my experience, which is supported by other psoriasis sufferers.

As with losing weight, if you become too consumed with the end result, you will not be available to the process. Trust that it is leading you to health and be patient. It is important to treat yourself with compassion. You deserve the very best in life, and old habits die hard!

According to Buddhist philosophy, we are here on Earth to experience happiness, not to suffer. We have to learn how to live without suffering; that is our task.

As the African people in South Africa say, "Nihambe kahle". Go well!

HEATHER J. FERRIS

PART ONE

WHAT IS PSORIASIS?

*Every belief is a limit to be examined and
transcended.*

JOHN C. LILY

You may be wondering if you have psoriasis. It would be a
good idea to have a medical diagnosis, but don't be surprised
if your general practitioner is not sure. Get another opinion
and know what you're dealing with. The following information is provided by the Canadian Psoriasis Foundation.

There are a number of different types:

- Guttate psoriasis is most common in children and young
  adults. The red patches look like drops, which appear on
  the trunk and limbs and sometimes the scalp. It often
  follows a strep throat infection or a cold, chicken pox,
  immunizations, trauma or antimalarial drugs.
- Erythrodermic psoriasis consists of patches that are more
  widespread. This is what I have.
- Pustular psoriasis, as the name implies, has pustules or
  blisters of pus that accompany the red patches.

- Inverse psoriasis is found in the armpit, groin, under the breast and other skin folds. It is often quite red and irritated.
- Psoriatic arthritis occurs in 5-10% of persons with psoriasis and is different from rheumatoid arthritis. It affects the last joint of the fingers and toes. Psoriasis accompanied by malformation of the nails may indicate this condition. I know this is present in my system.

You may be interested in how the skin works and what happens when psoriasis is present:

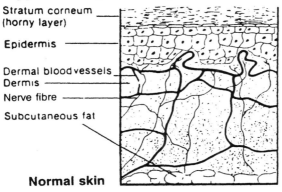

Stratum corneum (horny layer)
Epidermis
Dermal blood vessels
Dermis
Nerve fibre
Subcutaneous fat

Normal skin

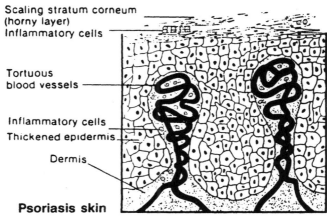

Scaling stratum corneum (horny layer)
Inflammatory cells
Tortuous blood vessels
Inflammatory cells
Thickened epidermis
Dermis

Psoriasis skin

HOW SKIN WORKS

Normal skin can be thought of as having two parts: a tough elastic inner layer called the dermis, and a thinner outer layer called the epidermis. The dermis is composed of the same sort of tissue as our ligaments and tendons. Within this layer lie the nerves and blood vessels that supply our skin, and also the tough fibres, known as collagen, that give healthy skin its suppleness and elasticity.

The epidermis is made up of lots of cells that are produced at its base (known as the basal layer). These move gradually up through the epidermis and become cells of the horny protective layer on the surface, and are ultimately shed. It normally takes about a month for a new cell in the basal layer to move up to the outer horny layer and drop off.

WHAT CHANGES OCCUR WHEN WE GET PSORIASIS?

Psoriasis affects the skin in several ways. The epidermis grows thicker so the psoriasis patch is slightly raised. This is caused because there is a huge increase in the basic number of cells within the epidermis. The cells themselves seem to swell, and fluid and blood cells accumulate in this layer. The whole epidermis becomes more folded than usual.

There are a number of changes that occur in the dermis. The blood vessels become much wider than normal, and the blood within them flows unusually rapidly. This explains why the patches are red and sometimes bleed. There are also a larger number of white blood cells than usual. Some of these move outwards and find their way into the outer layers of skin. In pustular psoriasis there is more inflammation and the collections of white cells form tiny abscesses, which account for the tiny pus spots patients have.

The cells in skin affected by psoriasis take about four days to move from the basal layer to the surface, while normal skin takes about twenty-eight days. Young cells are sticky which is why scale is produced.

The outer layer of our skin is usually an excellent protective barrier, keeping the body's fluids in and harmful substances out. But where there is psoriasis, water can escape anything from three to ten times faster than normal, so be aware of signs of dehydration, such as a dry mouth, decreased skin elasticity and general weakness.

Certain soaps and other chemicals against the skin can cause irritation. You may notice that nylon irritates the psoriatic skin. Some people using the Linotar/Exorex product cleared their psoriasis everywhere except their legs. When they stopped wearing nylons, their legs cleared up. Another patient found the only area that was resistent to treatment was her torso. She realized that she wore a nylon bathing suit which was inhibiting her healing.

One other effect of psoriasis is that the horny layer loses much of its pliability and toughness. As a result, cracks may develop, particularly on the hands or soles of the feet.

WHAT CAUSES PSORIASIS?

The cause is not known, although there is evidence that psoriasis has a genetic base, and this "defect" is inherited. When doctors suggested to me that psoriasis was genetic, my family could not identify anyone who had ever had it amongst their parents or siblings. It was interesting that just three years ago, my father developed patches on his leg at age seventy-seven. It cleared up after about six months. My niece at age sixteen developed psoriasis in response to successive throat infections. She had her tonsils removed and her lesions cleared up.

It seems that the right climate must exist for psoriasis to develop. This climate is connected to the state of the body's immune system. The immune system has been designed to maintain the body in a state of balance. The immune system will react to any abnormalities and rectify such imbalances where possible. We know the immune system has some enemies, which tend to weaken its functioning. These are stress, alcohol, high cholesterol, high blood sugar, aspirin, anti- inflammatories and so on. When the immune system is weakened, psoriasis can easily be triggered.

Stress relating to a traumatic experience is, more often than not, the trigger. The stress can also build up over a period of time and one event can be the catalyst. On reflection this is what happened to me.

When I was seventeen, I was already completing my first year at university. I was always tall for my age and very keen to keep up with my sister, who is eighteen months older than I am. I was an early reader and started grade one when I was five. People didn't realize that I was younger than my peers and I was not about to tell them. I was determined to 'keep up' socially although I was really not ready. I seemed to be proving to myself that I was okay, but I didn't feel okay. I felt, deeply, injustice of any kind. My rejection by my peers had been so painful and unjust.

I was always watching people and trying to understand what was going on. I was quite enmeshed in the lives of my parents and very sensitive to any disagreements. I took responsibility for the problems of others, a sign of co-dependency I recognize today. In 1964 I was taking a social work degree at the University of Cape Town in South Africa. My parents were building a house and living in an apartment temporarily. My sister and I stayed with a friend of the family, who was a dear woman, but she was a master at laying guilt trips. "You should be ashamed of yourself, messing around at university, when your parents could use your help financially. You should be out working." I was having great fun on the campus with sports, parties and social life. The course I was doing was not what I had anticipated and I was pretty scared that my well-meaning friend was right. I felt like a failure, but didn't want to give up the student life that held such social promise. I had also been trained to think that a university education was essential if you wanted to get anywhere in life......and my older sister was doing very well!

I never shared my feelings, so no one ever knew the workings of my psyche. I didn't admit my feelings even to myself. Outwardly, I was confident; inwardly, absolutely terrified. I have since discovered how stressful it is for the body when we don't express our feelings.

One event that really bothered me was when my parents gave my dog away without consulting me. She was barking a lot and bothering neighbours. My dog was very important to me. I didn't talk about it. Instead I was angry, hurt and confused about life. I kept things inside, something I have since learned is not useful to my health and certainly not necessary.

High stress brought about by low self-esteem, insecurity about my future and my family, loss of my dog and being unable to express my feelings, contributed, I believe, to the onset of psoriasis. I was forced to pay attention to my body, although doctors did not teach me how to do that. I lived in fear of the enemy, psoriasis, that had come to ruin my life.

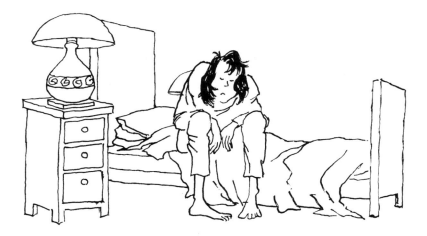

NOTES TO MYSELF

There is no greater illusion than fear, no greater
wrong than preparing to defend yourself, no greater
misfortune than having an enemy. Whoever can see
through all fear will always be safe

TAO TE CHING

Take some time now, or come back to this later. Reflect on
your life. You may want to continue in a separate journal.

What was happening in my life when the psoriasis first
appeared? _____

_____

_____

_____

_____

_____

_____

I was feeling _____
because _____
and _____

_____

_____

THE TREATMENT
MY STORY

*Within each of us lies the power of our consent to
health and to sickness, to riches and to poverty, to
freedom and to slavery. It is we who control these,
and not another.*

RICHARD BACH, *Illusions*

The psoriasis was diagnosed by our family physician, who
sent me to a dermatologist. I began one by one, the many
treatments familiar to psoriasis sufferers: cortisone, coal tar
and other sticky burning substances. They smelled awful and
stained my clothing. I would spend one day a week as an out-
patient at the hospital waiting first to see the doctor and then
for my prescription to be filled. The next stop was the physio-
therapist and the ultraviolet light treatment.

Summers were a bonus, as the beach and the sun were
favourites of mine. The lesions would recede in most areas,
because ultra-violet rays inhibit skin production, but I had
such body image problems, I would often not expose all areas
that needed treatment.

The constant flaking of my scalp and body generally caused me great embarrassment. I could not wear dark colours because I looked like I had severe dandruff. My most embarrassing moment occurred one night when I had gone to bed early. I was using the cortisone cream and I was wrapped in plastic from head to toe. My husband had been out with a friend, who came home with him for coffee. They had been drinking and the friend decided to come into our bedroom to wake me up to say hello. I had been lying there terrified that I would be seen and when he came in and switched on the light, the stress was almost more than I could bear. I dived under the covers. He probably doesn't even remember the incident and fortunately I have learned enough not to need plastic, nor to be held captive by the disease. If

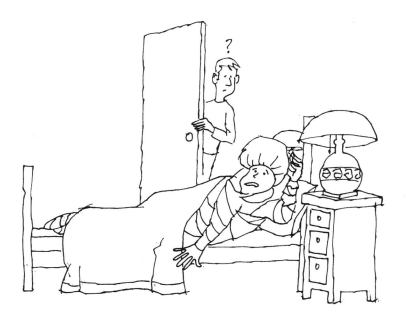

you have had the experience of wrapping your body each night you will understand how I felt.

Many people tried to help "cure" me with ointments and other concoctions their grandmothers had used for unknown skin problems. They meant well, but it became rather tiresome, particularly to a people pleaser! I'll never forget eating lecithin granules by the tablespoon, disguised in a jam sandwich while almost gagging, because I had been told that this was "the answer".

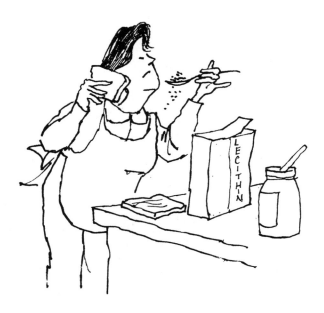

Then there was the brewer's yeast, vast quantities in orange juice, and the many herbal teas. All of the above have merit in the full scheme of things, but they all had one thing in common: they were described as the ultimate cure.

I do not believe there is an ultimate cure. Psoriasis is a wonderful example of the body saying, "I can't take this inner conflict any more. I will speak if you won't." Louise Hay, author of *You Can Heal Your Life* and other books, said that psoriasis is "The fear of being hurt. Deadening the senses and the self. Refusing to accept responsibility for our own feelings."

She suggests saying the following affirmation many times a day, "I am alive to the joys of living. I deserve and accept the very best in life. I love and approve of myself." Say it even when you least believe it. It works!

We are all looking for an immediate solution. Sometimes we find one and then realize later that there is a price to pay, maybe a health side-effect or some other disease. For example, the use of methotrexate seems to be beneficial for psoriasis short term, but can cause a problem in the liver; cortisone thins the skin. There is no quick fix, because all our parts are connected to one another; what affects one part of the system, affects another. We must pay attention to the needs of the body. If it is tired we should rest. If it is feeling stressed, we must take some action to relieve the stress. When we don't listen, diseases start to develop and we are not aware of them until they scream at us, as the red, angry lesions do with psoriasis.

As I reflect on my life since I developed psoriasis, I realize that certain things had a positive effect:

- I experienced success with diet and meditation while focusing on my husband's illness. My diet was not planned; it was all my body wanted given the emotional stress I was under. I ate yoghurt, fruit, nuts, muesli and salads.
- I lay in the sun, which offered at least seasonal relief.
- I had an interesting experience whilst teaching a group on self-caring. It was in winter. I was living in Australia and working with personal growth groups. The Self-Caring and Wellness group discussed self care needs in four sections: PHYSICAL, INTELLECTUAL, EMOTIONAL and SPIRITUAL.

Physical required us to have enough exercise, rest and good food, and to reflect on our reactions to foods (conscious eating).

We covered *intellectual* health, by deciding whether we were reading enough, taking the courses we wanted or meeting and talking with friends who stimulated our minds.

Emotional health included identifying our feelings and journal-writing about them to allow their expression. We also found other ways to express our feelings, like exercising, communicating more effectively or just having a good cry. Stress management exercises addressed both the physical and the emotional areas. One of the key elements in this course was experiencing fun and playfulness, which I discovered were really needed in my serious work-oriented life.

The *spiritual* needs were also considered. We spoke of the meaning of our lives and established some purpose in what we were doing. We used meditation practices to reflect deeply. It was a time of great learning for the group and for myself, as I put into practice most of what we were doing. It is one thing to think about life; it is another to live life. It was during these ten weeks that my skin cleared up totally even though it was winter at the time.

The sun and its healing had drawn our migration pattern from Edmonton's cold, to the warmer climate in California, then to Perth in Australia, an ideal psoriasis clearing climate. After four years in Perth, it seemed that it was time to move on, and I determined that this time, the climate was not going to dictate the destination. We returned to Canada.

I knew that it was time to trust that healing would continue regardless of the cold weather. I took into account all I had learned about my condition. I was now more practised at releasing my stress, where I had once kept it bottled up inside. I was aware of food as a trigger, but was not committed to doing anything about it. At times I would go off sugar, (just as a smoker quits for a while, then lights up again), but I would start again. I no longer drank alcohol, but that was not difficult for me to give up, as I only drank small quantities of wine on rare occasions.

In British Columbia, I was able to keep the psoriasis under control. This meant the lesions were still there, but not raised and angry. They were still there in winter covering most areas of my body. My skin was often itchy and I had many times felt compelled to scratch. This, of course, keeps the itch going and damages the skin, encouraging further psoriasis. I had discovered ways to deal with itching without scratching and I describe this in more detail in Section Two. I went through further major stress when my husband and I divorced and again when two of my children went to live with their dad in Australia for nine months. The psoriasis, although affected, was never as bad as it had been years before. I was much more aware of what was going on in my body and I took reasonably good care of myself.

Life was not all stress. I had many positive growth experiences. Five years ago I had the good fortune to be in a relationship in which I felt totally accepted in my body and this helped me to accept my physical self at last. I began to see myself in a new way.

A winter in which I had flu three times caused me to make a commitment to be healthy. If this meant getting rid of psoriasis, that would be great; if not, I would accept the disease and let it take its course. I was tired of focusing on psoriasis. It was, after all, just a means of the body expressing its pain.

I listened gently to my body each day. I walked when I felt the need, even when I was tired after a day at work. I found

I was refreshed afterwards. I heard my body rebelling against refined sugar. I made the commitment to eliminate sugar, dairy products, alcohol, eggs, citrus and red meat on advice given in a self-help guide, *Prescription for Nutritional Healing*, by James F. Balch, M.D. and Phyllis A. Balch, C.N.C.

I was also advised to add unsaturated fatty acids (primrose oil) to the diet as well as vitamin A, B complex, C, D and E. I decided after some trial that I would keep taking primrose oil each evening as well as blue-green algae which contains all the essential amino acids, beta carotene, all 8 vitamins, especially B-12 and is one of the highest sources of chlorophyll. I also take a calcium and magnesium tablet once a day.

I continued to exercise, have a monthly massage, write my journal and have regular laughs.

The lifestyle changes immediately caused weight loss and a sense of commitment. I felt energetic and alive. I began to meditate regularly. The psoriasis stabilised and the sun helped with the lesions. I firmly believe that the commitment to a healthy body helped the psoriasis and I was able to deal better with various emotional crises.

Winter came and the psoriasis returned, but not as severely as before. I was not concerned. Instead I was grateful that it was not as inflamed. I felt more at peace with my inner world.

A week before Christmas a package arrived for me from South Africa. My friend Margaret had heard a report on the success of a product, Linotar/Exorex (a mixture of coal tar and essential fatty acids extracted from banana skins). She had purchased some and sent it to Canada. My first reaction was to be grateful to her, that she had thought to help me. I also felt a certain reticence to try yet another remedy. I had worked hard to control the disease on my own and there was a part of me that wanted to complete the process. As I was contemplating this I heard, in my head, the voice of Noel, a psychotherapy trainer in Australia, who used to see how hard I worked at my personal growth. She said, "Heather, life doesn't have to be this hard."

Remembering this, I thought, "Maybe this has been sent to me to complement what I have already done." I decided to use it and, after four days, I noticed a remarkable improvement. After three weeks, from a body that had lesions covering eighty percent, on arms, legs, buttocks, torso, neck and around the hairline, there were only a few lesions on my shins! "Thanks Noel. Life doesn't have to be this hard!"

Though I celebrate the product Linotar/Exorex, I am aware that it is not only the product doing the work. If I want the psoriasis to go into remission, I must continue to listen to my body and take action to be healthy.

The real bonus from my journey in healing is the internal peace that I feel, and this seems to be growing and affecting all that I do. I am really grateful for what I have learned in my life.

NOTES TO MYSELF

Since the psoriasis first developed, I noticed an improvement
when _____

_____

_____

_____

_____

_____

Treatments (medical and non-medical) I have used that help
are _____

_____

_____

_____

Treatments I have used that I feel uncomfortable about are

_____

_____

_____

_____

DIET

"When you wake up in the morning, Pooh," said Piglet at last, "What's the first thing you say to yourself?" "What's for breakfast?" said Pooh. "What do you say Piglet?" "I say, I wonder what's going to happen exciting today?" said Piglet.

Pooh nodded thoughtfully, "It's the same thing," he said.

BENJAMIN HOFF, *The Tao of Pooh*

I hesitate to use the word diet, because it conjures up deprivation. You can't eat this or that, and you consider yourself a social outcast. We are socialized to want to be like everyone else, even when our body types are so different.

The body is a fantastic machine. If we learn to listen, we get all sorts of advice. I generally get heartburn from smoked products, yet I eat them because I like the taste! Sugar has, for a long time, caused me to become quite hyper inside and I feel really bad about myself when I get out of control with my sugar eating. I found that I had to eliminate refined sugar from my diet as I was unable to discipline myself to occasional use. If there was a dessert, it was really difficult for me to stop at one helping particularly if there was chocolate. Now I don't crave sweets or chocolate at all.

Pay attention to cravings. They tend to encourage us to be out of balance, out of control. Try eliminating these foods and eating something else. When I first developed psoriasis, I craved oranges. It may be that my immune system needed vitamin C, but my skin did not need citric acid. I did not know that then.

John finds that eating strawberries triggers his psoriasis. He doesn't notice it immediately, although some people do. It may be a couple of days later, that he notices the psoriatic lesions are inflamed. Others report reactions to citrus fruits, pork (bacon particularly), tartrazine, colourants and flavourings. One of the biggest enemies of psoriasis is alcohol, according to most research. Coffee and tea are often problems. If you drink them, try going without for a couple of days and see if you notice a difference in your skin. We are all different and we must listen to our own bodies.

High cholesterol levels block the transformation of essential fatty acids into the substances that support our immunity. When the intake of fatty foods is kept low and the cholesterol level is kept under control, our bodies have a much easier chance to overcome the psoriasis.

Pegasus Dermasearch, the company that makes the Linotar/Exorex products maintain that a healthy immune system is critical to the healing of psoriasis. This is probably true for all healing. Our bodies are sensitive to certain foods, even some that are nutritious. If there is some allergic reaction, our immune systems must work harder. Testing can help us determine which foods stress our body's immune system. It is useful to know whether we have a yeast overgrowth, which will also tax the immune system. Once we know our sensitivities we can eat with awareness. This does not mean we deprive ourselves. If I am sensitive to wheat, I will not eat many portions of wheat in a week.

The digestive and elimination system is connected to the skin. Foods that are difficult to digest could result in stress to the skin, since it is an elimination organ. Drink six to eight glasses of water a day to flush out toxins.

It is not useful to become obsessed by diet, because we become out of balance and stressed. We must, however, be conscious of what we put into our bodies and how our bodies respond to foods.

NOTES TO MYSELF

I eat the following portions of food in a week:

Meats (list red, chicken etc.)

Dairy products (list)

Vegetables (list)

Fruits (list)

Fats

Grains and Beans (list)

Snacks and desserts

Beverages/drinks

_____

_____

Foods, drinks I crave

_____

_____

Foods, drinks I am sensitive to

_____

_____

My eating habits can be described as (I eat too much, I eat irregularly, I eat on the run, healthy etc.)

_____

_____

I sometimes feel the following emotions around food

_____

_____

I will change my eating habits by

_____

_____

_____

_____

_____

_____

_____

THE MIND AND THE BODY

Wellness is the integration of body, mind and spirit —the appreciation that everything you do, and think, and feel, and believe has an impact on your state of health.

JOHN TRAVIS M.D. & REGINA RYAN,
The Wellness Workbook

LIVING IN YOUR HEAD

Our society has really valued people who are smart, educated and motivated thinkers. Many men (because of their social conditioning) describe how they are feeling by thinking about it, "Given this set of circumstances, how should/would I be feeling?"

I would often describe myself as someone whose spirit is ahead of her body.

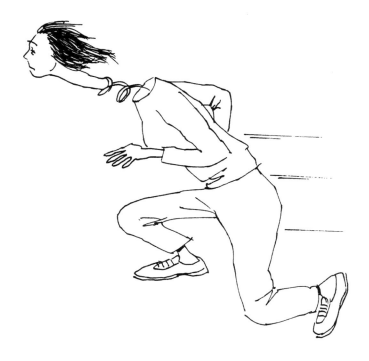

I had so many ideas and became involved in so many projects, my body had difficulty keeping up. I saw having so much enthusiasm for everything as a skill. I realize now that yes, I have a fertile imagination, and also a great disregard for the needs of my body. I never had respect for my body, so I focused on my mind. I believe now that psoriasis was one way for my body to scream for attention. Unfortunately, what I did was to focus on the psoriasis and not the body as a whole. The psoriasis was so unpleasant, that I blamed my body and its inability to cope. I developed a belief system that said my mind had control over my body, so all I needed to do was to develop enough mind control and the psoriasis would be beaten.

It is with great respect that I can now say, "My body is a very precious, necessary part of my life."It is my teacher, constantly communicating with me. I have so much to learn. My body teaches me about cause and effect. What I put into it is either digested with ease or with difficulty. My body gives me feedback such as gas, pain, sweating or vomiting if it is in distress. If I eat too much I feel uncomfortable. If I am not eating enough, I feel hungry, weak or dizzy.

My body also houses my emotions, which affect the functioning of my body. Anger for some manifests as a sore stomach or diarrhea, for others as a headache and for me as itchy skin or tense neck and shoulder muscles. If I am not aware of my body, I may just think about what is going on in my life and keep myself awake with the thoughts that go around and around in my head. The negative feeling states can be worked through the body much more quickly than through the head. You may find the breathing exercises in Section Two useful.

The body also lets me know what stress is on board. If I have a stiff neck, tight jaw or shoulders, it is generally not just the state of my body, but something going on in my mind. If I recognize the body stress and ask myself what I am worried about, I have the opportunity to work through the problem and relax the body at the same time.

Fear comes from either the past or the future. We are either regretting past events or fearful of the unknown. The only thing we can really have control over is the present. I find the acronym F. E.A.R. useful in understanding what fear really means.

F antasized

E xperience

A ppearing

R eal

So, we are projecting into the future. We have no evidence that our projection is true, although we sometimes make it come true.

The body deals only in the present, so if we are aware of our bodies as much as possible we will live far more in the present and experience greater peace. How many times has my mind been elsewhere and I've kicked my toe, even broken it, and come back to the present with a jolt, because I wasn't paying attention?

The mind takes control at great cost to the body. A business man was telling me recently that he is not aware of his psoriasis until the end of the day. When he gets home at night he is suddenly aware of how itchy he is. When we are not balanced we pay the price at the end of the day for pushing ourselves. I can really identify with this way of surviving. In the past I would push through an incredible amount of work with no thought to my own needs, be they bathroom needs or eating needs, or the need for a short rest. When the project was over and I allowed myself to relax, the psoriasis would get inflamed and itchy. The body had been on overload and totally disregarded.

When we take short breaks and listen to the needs of the body, it is possible to stay clearer, be more focused and to accomplish better work in less time. We have to give up the notion that someone racing from one place to another with furrowed brow, saying, "I haven't got time to stop. I am so busy," is actually productive.

Health is a choice and it can be our choice if we change our self-talk to reflect what we expect from our bodies. Mine goes like this, "I have a strong, healthy, beautiful body." I have said it so many times and resisted telling people about my ill-health, that I now believe it. I still get aches and pains, but I don't see them as ill-health, rather as signals telling me to change my eating or my exercising to accommodate the needs of my body.

Experiment the next time someone asks you how you are doing, and say, "Really busy," and then think of all that you are involved with. Be aware how that makes you feel. Another time say, "My life is great. I'm healthy and happy and I have a lot going for me." Now check your body reaction. The other reality is that most people are not wanting to hear about your busy-ness and fatigue. I am not suggesting you lie about how you are feeling and say the perfunctory, "Fine", but rather focus on what is going well. This really works for me. No matter how busy I am, I don't need to reflect on it because it drains more energy out of me.

Another way to conserve energy is not to replay the negatives of the day. Recently, I came out of a particularly disturbing meeting quite disenchanted with some of my colleagues. My first response on returning home was to call someone who had been at the meeting to commiserate. It took great willpower not to, knowing well that I would have been drawn even further into negativity by the end of the call, and I'd have taken her down with me. If you are angry it is important to do something to change the situation or tell the person concerned. If this is not possible or worthwhile, write in a journal and then let go.

Remember the wisdom in the Serenity Prayer: "God grant me the serenity to accept the things I cannot change, the knowledge to change the things I can, and the wisdom to know the difference."

NOTES TO MYSELF

Things that cause me stress in my life are ....because

_____

_____

_____

_____

_____

_____

_____

Underline those you think you can change. Star those you don't think you can deal with yourself. Write a list of those which are really not your problem and draw a helium balloon attached to each one. THEN IN YOUR MIND LET THEM GO!

_____

_____

_____

_____

_____

_____

_____

_____

REVIEW

- Pay attention to your body: the breathing and the signs of pain or discomfort in muscles or organs.
- Pay attention to the food you eat and eat with awareness, slowly, with gratitude and never when excited, angry or sad. Consider the effect foods have on your body. Are you reacting in a negative way to certain foods? Try different foods on their own if you are not sure. Drink six to eight glasses of pure water every day.
- Exercise with awareness, paying attention to the messages from the body. Feel the energy moving through the body as you build up your stamina. Exercise with joy, not grim determination, and feel the benefit to the body.
- Pay attention to your thoughts, because they have great power. "What I think, I am." If I think I'm stupid, my brain will act as if it is true. If I say, "I can't do this," I will most likely have difficulty. The past and the future are out of our hands in this moment. Our health is nurtured by love, not fear.
- Take action in your life to change situations that are not happy. The more you risk, the less you will fear.
- Ask for help or support when you need it.
- Take time each day to be quiet and relaxed. Begin and end the day reflecting on things you are grateful for in

your life. Include in this the positive changes you are making.

- Process your thoughts, actions and emotions through the use of a journal or artwork. Find out your motivation; be honest with yourself even when it hurts. Always question whether your actions are for the good of self and others.
- Play, laugh and have fun in your life: a belly-laugh releases our need to control.
- You are captain of your own ship; take responsibility for your life.
- Let go the need to control and trust that you will get all the help you need if you are awake.

The following tips are courtesy of the Canadian Psoriasis Foundation:

- Keep your weight down.
- Monitor alcohol intake.
- Expose skin to sunlight, but do not let it burn.
- Protect yourself against skin injuries.
- Avoid irritations to the skin such as plucking eyebrows, getting soap under a ring, wearing tight shoes, shaving legs or using harsh chemicals and cosmetics.
- Maybe try a humidifier in your home, especially when the air is dried out by central heating.

- Protect yourself from exposure to strep throat infections.
- Keep your skin moist with a moisturizer.
- Avoid exposing your hands to detergents if you have psoriasis on your hands. Try wearing cotton gloves under rubber gloves while washing dishes.
- Itching can sometimes be reduced by keeping the skin moist. Cold water will also help. Also full-strength apple cider vinegar used in bath water can help.
- When using a tar product use a downward stroke in the direction the hair is growing.

HAVE FUN IN YOUR LIFE. PSORIASIS, AND MOST OTHER DISEASES, GET FED BY THE 'POOR ME' VIBRATIONS!

NOTES TO MYSELF

_____

_____

_____

_____

_____

_____

_____

_____

_____

PART TWO

The body and mind need retraining. It is possible to quieten both down, even in a busy world. It is also possible to change our thinking and conditioning in order to de-stress our bodies. If we are willing to commit some time every day, we will notice an amazing difference in our lives, including better health, relationships and ability to work and enjoy ourselves.

The following exercises can help us heal:
The Full Breath
Quietening The Body And Mind
Dealing With Itching
Journal Writing
Healing The Heart
Meditation
Who am I?
Developing Gratitude
Inner Smiling

Wellness is the loving acceptance of ourselves.

THE FULL BREATH

Air is the first food of the newborn.
EDWARD ROSENFELD

Sit or stand with your spine straight, preferably in front of a mirror. Inhale and watch your shoulders. Do they rise? Try it again keeping your shoulders relaxed.

Now place your fingertips on your chest and feel the chest rise and fall as you breathe. Relax the shoulders as you do this.

Place you fingertips on your rib-cage and again experience the rising and falling of the ribs while the shoulders remain relaxed.

Take your fingers and place them gently on your belly and inhale, feeling the belly rise easily as you breathe. You may find difficulty with this breath. That is okay. Try lying down and relaxing. Feel your shoulders move away from your ears. Breathe into the abdomen. Don't try too hard. It will take time and practice. Allow the breath, don't force it. It is helpful to sigh as you exhale. Really let go.

It is quite common for us to shallow-breathe, because we tighten our chests, stomachs and lower abdomen when we are tense. The air just can't get in after a while! If you watch a baby breathing, you see the whole body rising and falling easily. Keep practising and you, too, will body breathe. The benefits to the body are a release of tension, a letting go.

Be aware of your breathing during the day. Are you holding your breath when under stress? If someone gets angry with you, what happens to your breath? If you get a fright, what do you do? When I started this practice, I wrote the letter "B" on strips of paper and left them where I would see them, at work, in my car and at home. This would remind me to pay attention to my breathing.

At the beginning of any situation that may cause anxiety, such as writing a test or saying something that is difficult to say to someone, take a deep breath and release it before you proceed.

It is useful to add the words, "Let go," as you exhale. This can be said out loud or in your mind. We have held on to much anxiety in our lives, including unexpressed emotions and words; our bodies have had enough. The body 'blows up' either through mental or physical illness or anger. Psoriasis is a perfect example of the body's inability to take any more stress. We just 'break-out'.

QUIETENING
THE BODY AND MIND

A full body relaxation and visualization of health.
This will take about thirty minutes.

Lie on a mat on the floor. Place a cushion under your knees to help protect your lower back. Make sure you will be warm enough. Be comfortable or you will not relax completely. Close your eyes gently. Your arms should rest at your sides or across the abdomen. This is not an opportunity to go to sleep, although the practice of relaxation is helpful in bed if you are having difficulty sleeping.

Breathe in easily. Be aware of your breath as it enters and leaves your body. Does it go into your chest, within your rib-cage or your belly area? Just be aware of it as it goes in and out. Be an observer, just watching the breath coming in and going out, in and out. It is sometimes helpful to imagine the breath having a colour. As you breathe in, watch the colour go into and through your body. As you exhale, breathe out any toxins, including stress. You may notice the exhalation is a different colour. Some people see it as grey or black; it doesn't matter. Breathe effortlessly and stay present. Don't allow yourself to drift off. Breathe in and out...... in and out.

Now that you are breathing easily, turn your attention to your shoulders and neck area. Do you feel any tightness? If you do, say to yourself, "Let go," on the exhalation and feel the tension leaving your body. Take your time breathing in and out easily and effortlessly. Do the same with your jaw, letting go of any tension........ and your facial muscles... your brow........ your head. Imagine that you are breathing healing, life-giving energy into each area and letting go of toxins and stress with each exhalation.

Move your attention to your arms and hands and breathe in nourishment, breathe out tension; just in and out, in and out......... Take your time. Next, focus on your chest and diaphragm. Include the heart and lungs, and feel the goodness filling each organ with the life force, and let go of everything not needed for optimum health. Continue this process slowly, watch every breath coming and going, in and out as you move into a deeper place of relaxation. Continue to the stomach and the elimination system, inhaling, exhaling, in and out........ letting go.

Breathe into the spine, feeling the movement of the vertebrae and the nerves from the tailbone to the brain, loose and easy, letting go of tension on each exhalation. Do this until you feel relaxed, breathing in and out.

Breathe into the reproductive area, gently release and relax. Observe the ease with which you allow the breath to move through you, bringing nourishment and letting go. You are perfect in this very moment.

Bring your attention to the buttocks being held by the floor or chair supporting you. You don't have to do anything. Now the legs, starting with the thighs, let go of any tightness.......... then the knees, they do a wonderful job supporting, allowing the body to be active......... remember to breathe and let go on the exhalation....... now the calves........ the ankles........ the feet. They each support us in our day-to-day lives. Take time right now to be gentle and appreciative of your feet.

Now the largest organ of the body, the skin. Breathe in to this wonderful supportive organ, that not only keeps all our parts together, but eliminates toxins and acts as a warning system that alerts us to the stresses of the body and the mind. It needs our love and nurturance. The skin does not cause psoriasis: it comes from the inner unrest, both physiological and psychological. Allow the skin to rest right now. If you are finding any irritation, do not respond by scratching or moving: that is a habit. Breathe in and out, watching the breath bring in healing and quietness and exhale anything that isn't needed. Keep doing this until you feel quiet and at peace.........................

Now allow yourself to imagine very comfortable surroundings, a place where you feel really safe and relaxed. This may be a place you've been, or a place you create right now. Use all your senses. What do you see (or feel you see)? What are the colours and shapes? Are you alone, or is someone there with you? Take your time, look around......... What sounds do you hear? Listen carefully allowing the sounds to be there, whatever they are............. What smells do you smell, or might you smell in this special place? Just flow with whatever comes.......... Reach out and touch things and feel the textures as you have this experience........... Can you taste anything? .... What feeling do you have about being there?

Now allow an image of yourself to rise up in front of you. Notice that your skin is beautifully soft and smooth........ disease-free. Notice what is happening in your mind. If you are disagreeing with the healthy vision, breathe and let go. Say: "It's okay to be healthy," and gently bring yourself back into the vision you are creating. Take as much time as you need to get a clear vision of yourself. Know, too, that with practice it will come. Say some affirmations at this time.

For example:

- I am enjoying a fit, healthy body. I am full of radiant good health.
- I love every part of myself, especially my skin.

- I am totally in control of my own healing. I allow that to happen now.
- I give thanks for the changes that are happening in my life, all the time, as I open myself up to healing.
- I love and approve of myself. I am enough.

Take as much time as you need. Embrace the vision of yourself if you feel able. Feel the love that is available to you at any time of the day or night. Remember you can come back to this same place whenever you wish. For now, say goodbye and be aware of this feeling of relaxation and peace. Bring it back with you.

Become aware of your body once again and focus on your breathing. When you feel ready, very gently open your eyes. Move slowly, stretching your arms and legs, wiggling your toes and your fingers. Be aware of how your body is feeling; get used to the feeling of being relaxed.

Get on with your day quietly. There is no hurry; be gentle with yourself.

This exercise is best done once a day, or twice if possible. Don't rush through the body: rushing is a sign the mind is not valuing the process. You are in charge and your body needs your help. We are not only healthier as we become less stressed, but also more productive. Remember, relaxation is not only a way of getting to sleep, it is a way of training the body to let go of tension. (A tape containing this exercise can be purchased. See ordering information at the back of the book.)

Remember your vision of a healthy, lovable you and take it with you as you go about your day. The real benefit comes when we are aware of our bodies as we go through the day. Sitting in a meeting with shoulders hunched and jaw clenched, or noticing my skin covered in psoriasis does not make me more accessible to my job, nor to my colleagues and certainly not to my family. I have noticed that people in a busy world are sometimes uncomfortable with my lack of tension. Some have made comments like, "You must have an easy life, you're always so calm." Initially I wanted to respond by justifying how hard I was working. Now I smile and feel good inside that people are noticing a difference. I am not always calm, but I do notice what is happening and take steps to relax.

DEALING WITH ITCHING

Many psoriasis sufferers experience itching. If you give it power, it can drive you crazy.

WHAT IS AN ITCH?

Itching is thought to be caused by very mild stimulation of pain nerve endings. There are a few very sensitive free nerve endings that respond to extremely light touch. It is possible that they carry the itch sensation. It is also possible to cause an itch sensation by merely thinking about a situation that has caused an itch in the past. The neurons in the brain recall the memory and the stress around the memory, the same way that a memory of a horrifying event causes us to become tense.

WHAT HAPPENS WHEN WE SCRATCH?

We cause mild, and sometimes not so mild, damage to the cells causing a further response from the nerve endings which intensifies the more we scratch. If we get too vigorous, the itch is replaced by pain. At this point we no longer feel the need to scratch and we are sometimes heard saying, "Well, the pain is worth it, at least I'm not scratching anymore!"

The reality is that the damage we have caused allows more psoriasis lesions to develop and so the cycle continues.

USING ITCHING AS A MEANS TO PRACTISE SELF-CONTROL

Remember that the mind is in charge of our responses. We want to quieten the mind and use it as an observer rather than a reactor. As you feel the itch sensation on your skin, focus on your breathing. Be aware of the breath going in and out, use the words 'in' and 'out' if you are having difficulty focusing. Keep your attention on your breath, not on the itch.

Once you feel a little more at peace, take your attention to the itch itself. Be aware of the actual sensation. *Do not respond by scratching*. Say to yourself, "Mild pain" and close your eyes observing what is going on in your body. Resist the urge to itch. It will pass, and you will emerge as captain of your ship. Sometimes a very gentle massaging of the area, thinking gentle, loving thoughts will also ease the itch. It is a great lesson in responding with gentleness rather than irritation. Psoriasis sufferers are often not loving of themselves.

Please note: It can never be emphasized enough that this is not an easy process. It is possible to make these changes if you are ready to make a commitment to change. If you find yourself reverting to scratching, instead of getting down on yourself, just say, "Start again," and be glad that you are noticing what you are doing. This is the first step in the change process.

JOURNAL WRITING

When we drop our masks with one another, we have a feeling of connection, of being truly known.... Before I can allow you to know me, I must risk knowing myself.

KAY LEIGH HAGAN,

A Journalkeeping Workbook for Self-Intimacy.

Journal writing is, in my opinion, one of the most useful ways to deal with something that is worrying us. Psoriasis and other diseases are made worse by the issues that we bury inside. It is important for our health to constantly release anything toxic, be that food or waste, anger, fear or resentment. We may choose to see a counsellor or talk with a good friend. Counsellors cost money, friends sometimes get tired if we are too needy. The journal is a private time just by ourselves. It can be confidential if kept in a private place. The fear that someone will read it sometimes becomes an excuse not to write. It costs nothing except the pain that has to come up before we can release it.

If you are familiar with this process, bear with me as I go over the basics. Later I will be describing a few specific exercises for you to try.

Journal writing is 'free writing'. Forget all the rules about writing you learned at school; the form and spelling do not matter. All that matters is that you are as honest with yourself as you can possibly be. This process will help you find out your truth so you may sometimes be surprised by what you write. Are you ready? You will need some paper, lined or plain, and a pen or pencil. Make sure you have at least half an hour set aside in a place where you will not be disturbed. I like to have a book that I keep specifically for my journal writing. It is interesting to reflect back on the different stages we go through in our healing.

Now to begin, take a deep breath and release. Sit comfortably, pick up your pen and start to write.

It may be that you can't start writing. You may wonder how to express yourself. As you think, so you must write, even if it means writing, "I can't write this down; I don't know what to say; I hate writing; this won't do any good; I feel stupid writing this down."

It is important to say how you are feeling. If I was very angry about a relationship, I might start like this: "I hate him. He lied to me. I trusted him. Why couldn't he tell me what was going on? I am so mad. I feel like a fool. Everyone else knew what was going on except me. That's really the worst: I feel a fool. Well, my friends don't think I'm a fool. They see him for who he is. He'll have to live with his conscience and that's not my problem ...."and so on, maybe coming to a place of sadness, "I feel really sad that the loving times with him are over. I know I'll get over it and it is obviously best in the long run. Right now I really miss him."

Keep writing until you feel finished for the moment. You will pick up on the issue again, but for the present let it go. I remember writing my journal to sort out my confusion about using methotrexate. The dermatologist had basically told me not to be 'stupid': methotrexate was definitely the best way to go. I had doubts, so, I started to write in order to find clarity. After I had listed reasons why the doctor should know what he was talking about, I described my intuitive feelings and my fears: ".......I am afraid that this drug will poison my system, damage my liver or something else. I also don't believe this deals with the cause of psoriasis. I feel so ignorant and out of control. I don't trust that this doctor has my best interests at heart. I really need people to care about me before I trust them................"

By the end I knew I needed more information about the drug. A friend researched methotrexate in the medical library and gave me the findings. When I read the information I became clear. I had known all along, but I needed verification to help my confidence in making my decision.

USING DIALOGUE IN JOURNAL WRITING

The dialogue method can be used to deal with a relationship with either a person or a disease. What we seek to accomplish is more understanding about the situation. Always take the time to relax and be comfortable. It may seem pretty weird to be talking to parts of your body. You may also be surprised at the responses you get. The process is similar to that of using an empty chair if you are practising a difficult conversation. You pretend the person is there. What you are doing in this dialogue is imagining that the skin can talk.

Dialogue with my skin may look something like this:

Me: Why do you have to look so ugly and itch?

Skin: I can't help it. It's what you put inside me that causes this disease.

Me: What am I putting inside? I eat healthy food.

Skin: It's not just the food, although that is important; it is all the worrying you do. It's not easy trying to adjust to all the toxins that are being created. My job is to eliminate toxins. Also, you have a bit of a problem with your sweat glands. They are not helping me enough. Remember, I am not the psoriasis. My cells can't perform properly when they're on overload.

Me: I guess you're right, but what can I do about it. I'd like to help, but what can I do?

Skin: I'm not the resident psychologist, but I hear that you take on too much and you don't let go of enough. If you could go through a day balancing that, it might help me out.

Me: I know you're right. The problem is, I feel for everyone and want to make it better, but I think that sometimes I am not doing what is right for myself. For example, what about diet?

Skin: Yes, about the sugar. It drives me wild. You need to listen to the messages all of us in the body are giving you as you take in food.

Me: Yes, the sugar one is hard for me to give up. I know I need to do it. Dairy products are another group of foods to think about. ....and so on.

Now, maybe you're thinking, "This is crazy". But, if it works, do you care? And it is helpful. You are your own healer. The more you recognize that all the answers are within you, the sooner the healing will begin.

Try a dialogue right now:

_____

_____

_____

_____

_____

_____

_____

_____

HEALING THE HEART

Things are not always the way they seem. Our feeling may be anger, but if we do some self-exploration we find that underneath anger is always fear or sadness. If we persist in being angry and not acknowledging the underlying feelings we do not heal. In fact we continue to chase people away instead of getting the support we need. Men have traditionally had more encouragement to stay angry rather than admit their vulnerability. They have also died sooner than women, who have traditionally expressed their sadness.

A journal process that helps to get beneath the surface emotion and heal the heart involves the following model called the Total Truth Process, used with permission from Jack Canfield, Self Esteem Seminars 1990:

There are six stages to go through. You may go through one and come back to it later. You may go through a few stages and then come back to one that you've already done. There are no rules, except to complete all stages eventually, if you want to experience healing of the heart.

1. ANGER AND RESENTMENT

Start your writing with one of the following:

> I'm angry that.........
>
> I hate it when...........
>
> I don't like it when.....
>
> I'm fed up with........
>
> I resent............
>
> I can't stand........

2. HURT

> It hurt me when............
>
> I feel hurt that..........
>
> I feel sad when............
>
> I feel awful about.........
>
> I felt sad when............
>
> I feel disappointed about.........

3. FEAR

> I was afraid that................
>
> I feel scared when...............
>
> I'm afraid that.................
>
> I get afraid of you when.........

4. REMORSE, REGRET, ACCOUNTABILITY

I'm sorry that...........

Please forgive me for.........

I'm sorry for...............

I didn't mean to.............

5. WANTS

All I ever wanted.........

I want you to............

I want/ed..................

I deserve.............

6. LOVE, COMPASSION, FORGIVENESS AND APPRECIATION

I understand that.......

I appreciate..........

I love you because............

I forgive you for...........

I forgive myself for...........

Thank you for................

I love you when...............

I love and appreciate myself, my body etc.

You don't have to use all of these sentence starters, only whatever seems right for you. Write as much in each of the six areas as you need. Try it now:

MEDITATION

*The only way to live a less tense life seems to be
by developing our mental and spiritual capacities.*
H.H. THE DALAI LAMA

The word, "meditation" may suggest, to some people, yogis sitting in isolation, legs crossed, maybe chanting, "OM".

Meditation for me is a state of being in which we lower our vibrations, in both the body and the mind. This induces calm. We are aware of the process as it takes place. We are not relaxing and going to sleep. Meditation often happens when we are sitting still, but it can easily be accomplished as we walk or swim, eat or contemplate.

In the West we talk of awareness; Buddhists speak about developing mindfulness. When we are mindful we are aware of thoughts, speech and actions. We are not fearful of the future or the past. We can't change the past and we really don't know the future and yet this is where we spend most of our time. Sit quietly for a moment and place your awareness on your breath as it goes in and out. Watch your thoughts. How easy is it to focus on the breathing without giving attention to those thoughts? Are you thinking of past events or are you anticipating the future? As you notice your attention leaving the breath, say, "start again," and go back to the breath. It sometimes helps to add the words 'in' and 'out'. This exercise improves your ability to be in the present time, in the moment, without fear. Practise for about ten minutes a day. You can practise while you are walking as well. This is called a walking meditation. Don't have a dog on the end of a leash when doing this; it doesn't work! Focus your attention on the ground about six feet ahead of you. As you step, say, "Right foot, left foot". Be aware of the foot as it touches the ground, feeling it supporting the body. If you notice your mind wandering, start again. Walk about 20 meters, turn and do it again continuously for about ten minutes. It is a way of training the mind to be present.

Mindfulness brings about inner peace and creates a vibration in the body conducive to healing. With practice we become more aware of our senses and they become intensified. We see more vibrant colours and become aware of the smells and sounds around us. We taste our food and feel the touch of our clothing, our feet on the ground and our connecting with others. This awareness allows us to listen to our bodies and our minds. It will help us to realize when we are eating something that is not right for our bodies, maybe a food or substance that is causing the psoriasis to flare up.

We will also become aware of the busy-ness of our minds and the self-talk that is also contributing to the toxicity in our bodies. Intuition will sharpen and we will become aware of the coincidences and flashes of inspiration that make life so much easier. We are wise beings by nature, aware of everything we need in life, but we have forgotten to listen. Instead, we have handed our power to doctors, teachers, lawyers and politicians.

This part of us that is wisdom is our spiritual nature, something many of us deny, perhaps because at some time we had a negative experience with religion. It is the part, I believe, that is connected to a higher consciousness, be that God or whatever name is comfortable for you. Our healing process is simple when we tap into our wisdom and spiritual consciousness.

There are many ways to meditate. There are a number of books on the subject. Find one that appeals to you and follow the instruction or attend a meditation class. Being in a group can be most helpful.

> True maturation on the spiritual path requires that
> we discover the depth of our wounds. As the
> Achaan Chah put it, "If you haven't cried a
> number of times, your meditation hasn't really
> begun."
>
> JACK KORNFIELD, A Path With Heart

WHO AM I?

This exercise is very useful in deepening your sense of who you are. You are more than your body, your mind and your personality. You can do this exercise by yourself or with a partner or friend with whom you feel comfortable.

If you are doing it on your own, find a quiet place where you can sit undisturbed. Ask yourself the question, "Who am I?" and write down whatever word comes to mind. Then ask again, "Who am I?" and keep doing this for about ten to fifteen minutes. If your mind is a blank write something you have written before. It doesn't matter. What does matter is that you continue, allowing yourself to be spontaneous. No-one need read this without your consent, so let yourself go.

If you are doing this with a partner, sit opposite the person. Set a timer for fifteen minutes. Look at your partner in a relaxed way. The first person asks the question, "Who are you?" You respond without writing it down. The person asking the question may not comment, laugh or prompt you. If you do not answer right away, it doesn't matter. Your partner should stay silent and give you time. If emotions like laughter, tears or feelings of discomfort come up, stay with them and breathe. They will pass. After the first fifteen minutes change partners. You will be amazed at how your responses deepen. For example: Most people at first say their name, then the various roles they take in their lives, like mother, worker etc. They move on to hobbies, recreation and interests. They move a little later into qualities like, a caring person, a person who values honesty, then on to aspirations for their life. The more you do it, the deeper it gets.

The ultimate goal of this exercise is to reach a better personal understanding of your purpose here on the planet. As we become more intimate with ourselves we can discover who we really are underneath all the societal and family conditioning.

Try it now:

I am _____

_____

_____

_____

_____

_____

_____

_____

DEVELOPING GRATITUDE

A very important key to developing this consciousness is to realize how very fortunate we are. Gratitude is an attitude that we can develop with sincerity. No matter how difficult our lives, there are many things that we have to be grateful for. The healing vibration does not come when we are negative and feeling sorry for ourselves. We have to raise this vibration by focusing on how fortunate we are. Try it right now. I am fortunate because

_____

_____

_____

_____

_____

_____

_____

_____

It takes discipline sometimes to stay focused. Our tendency when we are irritable or in pain, is to stay there. If you find your mind wandering back to your problem, say gently, "start again". I am really fortunate..........., I appreciate.......... and so on. Notice how you are feeling inside. Be aware of what I call the slowing down of the vibration. If you find you are getting excited: breathe and relax. This will put you back in control, instead of the adrenal system exciting all the organs in the body.

Our bodies have become accustomed to a variety of intrusions from an industrial lifestyle. The stresses and strains often lead to fearful bodies and minds. It will take a while, practising regularly, to create inner peace.

The development of the practice of meditation is most useful, but it is important to practise the basics before you move on to experiencing other things. Learning from an experienced teacher can be helpful. Like most things that are good for you, meditation requires perseverance and patience. It really is worth it.

INNER SMILING

This exercise is taken from, *The Attitude of Gratitude* by Donna Martin (used with permission).

Lie in a relaxed position. Start to scan your body by moving your attention gently and effortlessly through your entire body. Just notice whatever you're experiencing. Now rest your attention for a moment on your face and eyes. Begin to allow yourself to smile, just a little. Feel the beginning of the smile, the first movements and subtle changes, especially around the eyes.

Next, place your fingertips lightly on the solar plexus, the centre of the upper abdomen, just below the diaphragm. Let your fingers sense any changes that occur here when you smile. Now frown or grimace, then slowly smile again. Do you notice how the solar plexus 'smiles' too?

Move your attention back to your eyes and face and gently invite the smile to broaden. Do this as easily as possible, without any effort or strain. Imagine that this smile expresses genuine delight and appreciation, and that these qualities shine into any area where the smile is focused. Imagine the smile moving from the face into the inside and back of your head. Feel as if the smile moves down into your throat and the back of your neck. Pause in each location until you get a real sense of a smile in each place.

Whenever necessary, remember how the smile feels by going back to the eyes and the solar plexus. Slowly move the smile down into the shoulders... into the chest, the upper back... down the middle and lower back... into the belly. Let an inner smile move into all the internal organs: the lungs, the heart, the liver and kidneys, the pancreas and spleen, the intestines, the bladder, the reproductive organs.

Imagine the pelvic floor relaxing into a smile. Let the smile gradually move down the whole body into the legs and the feet. Come back to noticing the smile in your face, your solar plexus, your chest... Feel as if the smile moves into your arms and all the way down into your hands. Let this inner smile move through your whole body and let it rest in any areas you feel are in need of healing or appreciation.

After feeling your whole body smiling from the inside out, just rest for several minutes, noticing whatever you are experiencing.

(For more exercises to cultivate the Art of Appreciation contact Donna Martin Box 834, Kamloops, B.C. V2C 5M8.)

TREATMENTS FOR PSORIASIS

Extracts reprinted, with permission from the booklet, *Understanding Psoriasis*, published by the Canadian Psoriasis Foundation, 1994. This can be obtained for approximately $7.00 Canadian including shipping and tax. The address is Suite 500A, 1306 Wellington St. Ottawa, Ontario K1Y 3B2, telephone 1 800 265 0926 and fax 613 728 8913.

In the U.S.A. contact the National Psoriasis Foundation, 6600 SW 92nd, Suite 300, Portland, Oregon 97223. Tel. 503 244 7404 and fax 503 245 0626, for further information.

The new treatment that I obtained from South Africa is called *Linotar/Exorex* gel and conditioner. It is really easy to use, doesn't stain clothing much and doesn't have a strong smell. This non-prescription product is made from essential fatty acids found in the banana peel, which are mixed with coal tar. Possible side effects: tar can irritate the skin in some people. Try it on a small area first. Tar can make the skin dry, so this product comes with a compatible cream. Linotar/

Exorex is not at present available in North America, although registration is in process in Canada. For information about the product in Canada and the U.S.A. contact, Walt Bros. International Inc., 184 Tansley Road, Thornhill, Ontario L4J 4E7, Tel. 1 800 839 6739, Fax (905) 771 8315.

It can also be obtained directly from Pegasus Dermasearch, Pty. Ltd., P.O. Box 77218 Fontainebleu 2032, Transvaal, South Africa. You can order using a credit card by calling 011 27 11 792 9516. Your questions about psoriasis will be answered willingly. Remember the time difference!

Other tar products may be prescribed by your physician and tar-based shampoos can be found on pharmacy shelves.

A vitamin D3 analogue called calcipotriol, sold under the brand name of *Dovonex*, is an ointment to be applied twice daily. It is not for use by patients under eighteen years of age. It is a prescription product. Side effects: 20% of patients will experience stinging for the first few days of use. This normally subsides. You should not use more than 100 grams per week, unless authorized by your physician.

PUVA is the combined use of a long-wave ultra-violet light and a prescription medication called psoralen. Side effects in some patients include premature aging of the skin, nausea, itching, depression, dizziness, insomnia, headache, cold sores, increased incidence of squamous cell carcinoma, cataracts, immunosuppression, increased risk of genital cancer in men.

Cyclosporine is an immunosuppressive agent available for the treatment of psoriasis as Sandimmune. It is taken orally. Side effects in some patients include high blood pressure, abnormal kidney function, an increase in malignancies, stomach complaints, increasing body hair, swelling of gums, fatigue and flu-like symptoms.

Methotrexate is a drug that seems to offer relief. Always ask doctors to give you detailed information about possible side-effects. This and other drugs have potentially serious side-effects.

Cortisone ointments are often prescribed. Be aware that cortisone thins the skin.

Useful Herbs: dandelion, goldenseal, sarsaparilla and yellow dock. See *Prescription for Nutritional Healing* by James F. Balch and Phyllis A. Balch, Avery Publishing Group Inc., Garden City Park, New York, 1990.

Naturopathic Remedies: Consult a naturopathic physician for advice.

Please note that the above medical treatments only deal with the disease, not the whole body. Linotar/Exorex is the only product, in my experience, which is marketed in conjunction with a holistic approach to the treatment. The company provides healing clinics in South Africa, which provide a wonderful setting in which clients can, under the supervision of professional staff, relax and follow a treatment plan. For further information contact Pegasus Dermasearch (see above address).

Another therapeutic setting is found in Israel. Contact the Psoriasis Foundation for details about the Dead Sea Centre.

It is possible that once Linotar/Exorex is registered in Canada, similar residential clinics will be available here.

HELPFUL HINTS FROM PEOPLE WITH PSORIASIS

The following excerpts are from letters written by people with psoriasis indicating successful treatments:

"I am a twenty-seven year-old female. While my psoriasis cannot be described as severe, it developed quite rapidly over the last two years and was becoming very irritating to me. Various dermatologists were unable to help me, despite the prescription of countless medications. As my health plan at work covers the treatment of a naturopath, and I was getting desperate to control the psoriasis without the use of excessive amounts of drugs, I decided to visit one.

While I was initially very sceptical of the whole field of naturopathy, I have, after successfully controlling most of my psoriasis through it, come to believe that it does have some very sensible tenets. The treatment he prescribed fell into four general areas:

- diet and nutrition
- herbal supplements
- vitamin supplements
- stress management

While making these changes to my daily routine took some time, I began to see an improvement after one or two months. While I do not follow the diet religiously (I travel almost all week due to my job and it is fairly difficult to get all the requisite foods at times), I have made permanent changes to my eating habits (no more diet coke) and continue to take the supplements on most days. I also added n-acetyl-glucosamine (NAG) to the list of supplements I take and that seems to help a great deal as well, (when I run out of NAG my psoriasis flares up a little).

I believe there is room for both alternative and conventional methods in the treatments of psoriasis - however, it is my preference to be drug-free if I can, so the naturopathic approach has been great for me.

Diet:

- 6-8 glasses of pure water each day
- 80% of the diet from the fruit and vegetable group
- 20% from the grain and meat group

Avoid:

- all red meat except lamb
- all nightshade plants: tomatoes, eggplant, peppers, white potatoes, paprika, tobacco

- alcoholic beverages
- all fried foods, pizza, pop, sweets and pastries, sugary cereals, chocolate, gravies, wine or grain vinegars, & hot spices

Nutritional supplements:

- folic acid, vitamin A, vitamin E, selenium, zinc, flaxseed oil, fish oils."

S.M.

Please note: I suggest you consult a naturopath for more information.

"Our daughter was diagnosed with psoriasis when she was nine years. We decided to investigate alternative possibilities before we used what was prescribed. I took her to a naturopathic physician who took a full history and felt that her problem was with her liver, which could not detoxify her system properly, and so her skin was being affected. She was given a homeopathic remedy (a solution under her tongue), and took a beet leaf base naturopathic remedy for some months. Her psoriasis cleared up somewhat, but really improved when she went for photo treatments. She now keeps it under control using a coal tar soap, biojoba shampoo and taking an evening primrose capsule every night. Summer is not a problem, since she gets enough natural radiation. She has never had to return for light treatments (in three years)."

S.C.

If you, the reader, have helpful hints, please share them with others either through a newsletter or by writing to me. We have so much to teach one another. No one person is the expert. We each have our experience and it is all valid.

IN CONCLUSION

Whichever way you go, know that millions of fellow psoriasis sufferers are cheering you on. It takes courage to make life changes and even more courage to stick with them.

You may choose drug therapy, but do remain in charge of your healing. Listen to your body. Realize that you have the right to compassion and information from doctors and other health-care professionals. Find someone you feel comfortable with; maybe you already have.

There are many treatments out there, herbal and others. Write me if you have had success with any of them and I'll make the information available. The address is 510 Harlech Road, Qualicum Beach, B.C. V9K 1K6.

We often hear about the "heartbreak of psoriasis". It's a difficult disease to treat, without question, but I believe it only breaks our hearts if we allow it.

"I am not my body; I am not my skin; I am not psoriasis."

If people react to our condition, they are not reacting to us. More often their reaction comes from ignorance and fear. Be patient with them: educate them. Help them to recognize the person inside the psoriasis-inflamed, or psoriasis-encrusted body, who has feelings, and wants to be loved and accepted just like everyone else. If they choose not to understand, let go. It is not your problem. We must take care of ourselves. This is our job. If we don't, we pay for it.

Our bodies are sacred. They may not function, at times, the way we'd like, but they are doing the very best job they can under the circumstances. We must treat them with love. This means with kindness and compassion, as we would someone we hold dear. Love is an incredible healer. Go with love.

BIBLIOGRAPHY

I found the following books useful in my healing. There are many more. Browsing in a book store and having a title 'jump out' at you is often the best way to determine what will be helpful at any given time.

Bach, Richard. *Illusions.* Great Britain: William Heinemann Ltd., 1977.

Balch, James F. and Phyllis A. *Prescription for Nutritional Healing.* New York: Avery Publishing Group, 1990.

Canfield, Jack and Hansen, Mark Victor. *Chickensoup For The Soul.* Florida, U.S.A.: Health Communications, Inc., 1993.

Chopra, Deepak. *Perfect Health: The Complete Mind/Body Guide.* New York: Harmony Books, 1991.

Ferris, Charles. *A Small Gift.* Qualicum Beach B.C. Canada: Melville Publications, 1993.

———. *Twelve Dimensions.* Qualicum Beach BC: Melville Publications, 1988.

Gawain, Shakti. *Creative Visualization.* New York: Bantam Books, 1982.

Gibran, Kahlil. *The Prophet.* London: William Heinemann Ltd., 1926 (reprinted 1971).

Gyatso, Geshe Kelsang. *Buddhism.* London: Penguin Group, 1984.

Hagan, Kay Leigh. *Internal Affairs: A Journalkeeping Workbook for Self-Intimacy.* New York: HarperCollins, 1990.

Hay, Louise. *You Can Heal Your Life.* Carson CA: Hay House Inc., 1987.

Jampolsky, Gerald. *Love Is Letting Go Of Fear.* Berkeley CA: Celestial Arts, 1979.

Kornfield, Jack. *A Path With Heart.* New York: Bantam Books, 1993.

Martin, Donna. *The Attitude of Gratitude.* Kamloops BC: Cardinal Publishing, 1994.

————. *Beyond Coping: The Journey of Recovery.* Kamloops, BC.: Cardinal Publishing, 1994.

Mitchell, Stephen. *Tao Te Ching.* New York: Harper & Row, 1988.

Progoff, Ira. *At A Journal Workshop.* New York: Dialogue House Library, 1975.

Robbins, John & Mortifee, Ann. *In Search of Balance.* California: H.J. Kramer, 1991.

Ryan, Regina Sara & Travis, John W. *The Wellness Workbook.* Berkley CA: Ten Speed Press, 1981.

Silva, José & Stone, Robert B. *You The Healer.* California: H.J. Kramer, 1989.

Steinem, Gloria. *Revolution From Within: A Book of Self Esteem.* Boston: Little, Brown & Co., 1992.

Weissman, Steve and Rosemary. *With Compassionate Understanding: A Meditation Retreat.* Bangkok, Thailand: P. Samphanpanich Ltd., 1990. Wat Kow Tahm International Meditation Center, Ko Pahngan Island, Thailand.